AYURVEDA COOKBOOK

MAIN COURSE - 80+ Step-by-step Guide to increase your energy and heal yourself

TABLE OF CONTENTS

responsibility or blame be held against the publisher for any reparation, damages, or monetary loss due to the information herein, either directly or indirectly.

Respective authors own all copyrights not held by the publisher.

The information herein is offered for informational purposes solely, and is universal as so. The presentation of the information is without contract or any type of guarantee assurance.

The trademarks that are used are without any consent, and the publication of the trademark is without permission or backing by the trademark owner. All trademarks and brands within this book are for clarifying purposes only and are the owned by the owners themselves, not affiliated with this document.

Introduction

Ayurveda recipes for personal enjoyment but also for family enjoyment. You will love them for sure for how easy it is to prepare them.

HERB FRITTATA

Serves: *3*

Prep Time: *10*   Minutes

Cook Time: *20*   Minutes

Total Time: *30*   Minutes

INGREDIENTS

- 6 eggs
- 1 tbsp parsley
- some spinach leaves
- ¼ tsp salt
- a pinch pepper

DIRECTIONS

1. Preheat your oven to 350°F
2. Boil the spinach and then remove the water
3. In a bowl, whisk the eggs and add the spinach and the other ingredients
4. Put the mix into the oven for 20 min

Serves: *4*

Prep Time: *10*   Minutes

Cook Time: *15*   Minutes

Total Time: *25*   Minutes

INGREDIENTS

- a cup flour
- 2 cups water
- onion
- a pinch of salt

DIRECTIONS

1. In a bowl, combine the flour with water until it gets consistent
2. Chop the onion and combine it with the mixture
3. Spread your mixture on the frying pan and after 3 minutes, flip it over and there you have it

Serves: *2*

Prep Time: *5*   Minutes

Cook Time: *10*   Minutes

Total Time: *15*   Minutes

INGREDIENTS

- a cup quinoa
- a cup milk
- a cup water
- a pinch salt
- a sliced fruit

DIRECTIONS

1. Mix all the ingredients in a saucepan
2. After you get it to a boil, cover the top and let it sit until water is absorbed

Serves: *2*

Prep Time: *10*   Minutes

Cook Time: *15*   Minutes

Total Time: *25*   Minutes

INGREDIENTS

- a cup oats
- any fruits you like
- a glass water
- a glass milk
- sweetener or honey

DIRECTIONS

1. Combine the oats with water in a saucepan and let it boil
2. Drain the water and let it sit for 5 minutes and then and the milk
3. Slice your fruits and put them in a frying pan with some water and let them covered for 3 minutes.
4. Mix the oats together with the fruits and you are ready to serve

Serves: **2**

Prep Time: **10**   Minutes

Cook Time: **20**   Minutes

Total Time: **30**   Minutes

INGREDIENTS

- 3 tbsp raw coconut flakes
- 1 tbsp oil
- 1 cup oat flakes
- 1 tsp sugar
- 3 cups water

DIRECTIONS

1. Boil the water and add the oil and sugar
2. Over the boiling water, add the oats and stir until it gets soft and creamy
3. Top it with the coconut flakes and serve

Serves: *1*

Prep Time: *10*   Minutes

Cook Time: *5*   Minutes

Total Time: *15*   Minutes

INGREDIENTS

- 1 apple
- 1 tsp dry ginger
- 1 tbsp sugar

DIRECTIONS

1. In a saucepan add the sliced apple with 1 cup of water and let it boil with the sugar
2. Add the ginger and continue stirring
3. Served warm

Serves: **2**

Prep Time: **5**   Minutes

Cook Time: **5**   Minutes

Total Time: **10**   Minutes

INGREDIENTS

- 2 bananas
- 1 cup fresh cilantro
- 2 tbsp lemon juice

DIRECTIONS

1. Cut the bananas and add the other ingredients and mix them well, but gently and it is ready to be served

Serves: *3*

Prep Time: *5*   Minutes

Cook Time: *25*   Minutes

Total Time: *30*   Minutes

INGREDIENTS

- 3 apples
- 1 tsp cinnamon
- little butter
- 1 tsp rosemary

DIRECTIONS

1. Preheat the oven to 370°F
2. Arrange your sliced apples in a baking plate
3. In a pan, melt the butter and pour it over the apples evenly
4. Sprinkle the cinnamon and the rosemary on top of the slices. Put it in the oven for 30-35 minutes

Serves: *4*
Prep Time: *10*   Minutes

Cook Time: *15*   Minutes

Total Time: *25*   Minutes

INGREDIENTS

- 1 tbsp vinegar
- 1 tsp chili
- 1 tsp coriander
- 1 tbsp butter
- 1 cup ground corn
- a pinch salt

DIRECTIONS

1. Combine the coriander, chili, and salt in a bowl
2. In a saucepan, boil 1 cup water with salt and vinegar and pour it over the mixture
3. Add the ground corn and knead until it has a uniform texture
4. Create medium sized balls out of the dough and flatten it after your preference
5. Fry the dough in a frying pan with butter and serve it

Serves: **2**

Prep Time: **10** Minutes

Cook Time: **30** Minutes

Total Time: **40** Minutes

INGREDIENTS

- 1 cup rice
- a pinch pepper
- 1 clove garlic
- 1 tbsp butter
- 1 tsp dry ginger
- 1 pinch salt

DIRECTIONS

1. Fry the chopped garlic in a pot with butter and the dry ginger for 3 minutes
2. Add 3 cups water and let it boil
3. While stirring, add the rice and the other ingredients and keep stirring for 5-6 minutes
4. Reduce the heat to minimum and let it drain for 6 minutes

Serves: *2*

Prep Time: *8*   Minutes

Cook Time: *22*   Minutes

Total Time: *30*   Minutes

INGREDIENTS

- 1 cup rice
- 1 tsp cinnamon
- 3 pices figs
- 1 tbsp butter
- 1 pinch salt
- 3 cups water

DIRECTIONS

1. Heat a saucepan on low and add butter and chopped figs
2. After the butter has melted, add raw rice and stir for 4 minutes until the rice smells nice and it is full of butter
3. Add the figs and the rest of the spices and stir again for 2 minutes
4. Add water and let it boil
5. Cook for 12-15 minutes covered with a lid
6. Serve when ready

Serves: **2**

Prep Time: **5**   Minutes

Cook Time: **20**   Minutes

Total Time: **25**   Minutes

INGREDIENTS

- 1 cup rice
- 2 pinch salt
- 1 tbsp cilantro
- 1 clove garlic
- 1 tbsp butter
- 1 pinch salt

DIRECTIONS

1. Chop the garlic and fry it in a saucepan with butter
2. Add 2 cups water and boil
3. Add all the remaining ingredients and stir
4. Reduce the temperature and simmer for 12-15 minutes
5. Serve when ready

Serves: *3*

Prep Time: *10*   Minutes

Cook Time: *25*   Minutes

Total Time: *35*   Minutes

INGREDIENTS

- 2 tbsp nuts
- 1 tsp cinnamon
- 1 tsp butter
- 1 tsp any kind of syrup
- 1 cup milk
- 1 cup oats

DIRECTIONS

1. Grind the nuts and the oats together
2. In a saucepan, combine all the ingredients including the nuts and oats
3. Add the milk and let it boil while stirring
4. Lower the heat and let it sit for 10 minutes
5. Serve when ready

Serves: 2
Prep Time: *10*   Minutes

Cook Time: *30*   Minutes

Total Time: *40*   Minutes

INGREDIENTS

- 1 tsp cinnamon
- 2 pears
- 1 cup water

DIRECTIONS

1. Preheat the oven to 300°F
2. Place the sliced pears on a baking plate and fill the bottom of the plate with water
3. Sprinkle on top of the pears with cinnamon
4. Bake in the oven for 15-18 minutes

Serves: *2*
Prep Time: *5*   Minutes

Cook Time: *10*   Minutes

Total Time: *15*   Minutes

INGREDIENTS

- 2 bananas
- 1 tsp cilantro
- a pinch salt
- 1 tsp lemon juice

DIRECTIONS

1. Cut the bananas without the peel in any size you want
2. Sprinkle on cilantro, salt, and the lemon juice
3. Mix well, but gently

Serves: **2**

Prep Time: **5**   Minutes

Cook Time: **15**   Minutes

Total Time: **20**   Minutes

INGREDIENTS

- 1 cup semolina
- 1 cup milk
- 1 tbsp butter
- 1 tsp cinnamon
- 2 tsp sugar

DIRECTIONS

1. In a pan, dry roast the semolina for 3-4 minutes
2. Add the milk and stir constantly
3. Pour the cinnamon to the mixture and let it boil
4. Lower the heat and let it simmer 10 minutes
5. Serve hot

Serves: **4**

Prep Time: **10** Minutes

Cook Time: **20** Minutes

Total Time: **30** Minutes

INGREDIENTS

- 1 cup small flageolet beans(soaked overnight)
- 1 tsp ground coriander
- 2 tbsp butter
- a pinch salt
- a pinch dry ground ginger
- a pinch ground turmeric

DIRECTIONS

1. Blend the beans with 2 tbsp water until creamy
2. Add salt, turmeric, ginger, and coriander
3. In a pot, melt butter
4. Pour the creamy mixture in the pan and cook for 5-7 minutes and flip it over and let it cook for 3-4 minutes
5. Repeat step 4 until the mixture is finished

Serves: *4*

Prep Time: *15*   Minutes

Cook Time: *10*   Minutes

Total Time: *25*   Minutes

INGREDIENTS

- 1 cup milk
- 1 tbsp baking powder
- 3 eggs
- 1 tbsp butter
- 3 tbsp any syrup you like
- 1 cup pumpkin
- 1 tbsp sugar
- a pinch salt
- 1 cup flour

DIRECTIONS

1. Melt the butter and beat the eggs
2. Mix the dry ingredients and make a hole in the middle in which you pour the wet ingredients and then whisk well
3. Butter a waffle griddle and pour in the mixture
4. Cook the waffles 5-7minutes until soft and golden, pour over the syrup and serve when ready

Serves: 2

Prep Time: 5   Minutes

Cook Time: 15   Minutes

Total Time: 20   Minutes

INGREDIENTS

- 2 pinch cinnamon
- 1 tsp butter
- 1 tsp any syrup
- 2 tbsp oats
- 1 cup water

DIRECTIONS

1. Boil the water in a saucepan and add the rest of the ingredients and lower the heat
2. Cook until the oats are soft
3. Serve warm

Serves: *4*
Prep Time: *10*   Minutes

Cook Time: *30*   Minutes

Total Time: *40*   Minutes

INGREDIENTS

- 1 cup water
- 2 tbsp quinoa
- 1 pinch pepper
- 1 tsp butter
- 1 pinch salt
- ½ soy sauce

DIRECTIONS

1. Boil quinoa in water
2. Drain the quinoa and put it in a bowl
3. Place in the bowl the rest of the ingredients and mix well
4. Serve warm

SWEET POTATO WITH KALE AND BEANS BOWL

Serves: *2*

Prep Time: *10*   Minutes

Cook Time: *20*   Minutes

Total Time: *30*   Minutes

INGREDIENTS

- 2 cup beans
- 1 tsp coconut oil
- ½ tsp dry ground ginger
- 2 kale leaves
- a pinch salt
- 1 cup sweet potato

DIRECTIONS

1. Grate the potato and chop the kale
2. In a pan on medium heat add the coconut oil and place the kale, the sweet potato, and the beans
3. Boil and cover, cook for 15-20 minutes, stirring occasionally until tender
4. Serve when ready

Serves: *3*

Prep Time: *5*   Minutes

Cook Time: *15*   Minutes

Total Time: *20*   Minutes

INGREDIENTS

- 2 cup cauliflower
- 1 tsp coriander seeds
- 1 cup fennel bulb with stalk
- 2 tbsp pumpkin seeds
- 1 cup water

DIRECTIONS

1. Chop the cauliflower and the fennel
2. In a pan, cook for 2-3 minutes the pumpkin seeds on medium heat stirring constantly and set aside
3. In a saucepan add the rest of the ingredients and cover with a lid and steam on medium heat until the result is tender
4. Serve with the pumpkin seeds

Serves: *3*

Prep Time: *10*   Minutes

Cook Time: *20*   Minutes

Total Time: *30*   Minutes

INGREDIENTS

- 1 tsp chili powder
- 2 pinch coriander powder
- 2 pinch turmeric powder
- 1 pinch pepper
- 1 pinch salt
- 3 tbsp tofu
- 1 cup spinach
- 3 corn tortillas
- any vegetables you like (cilantro, carrots, lettuce, avocados, cucumber, salsa)

DIRECTIONS

1. Mix all the spices in a bowl
2. Drain well the tofu
3. In another bowl, mash the tofu and combine it with the spices

4. Heat olive oil in a frying pan on low heat and then add the tofu and start to fry it for 5 minutes

5. Add the chopped vegetables you have and stir for 5 more minutes and set aside

6. Warm the tortillas in another pan on low heat for 2 minutes

7. Serve the tortillas with the tofu mixture

Serves: *3*

Prep Time: *5*   Minutes

Cook Time: *10*   Minutes

Total Time: *15*   Minutes

INGREDIENTS

- 1 tbsp oil
- 1 tsp mustard seeds
- 2 tsp yellow split peas
- 1 tsp black lentils
- 1 tsp chili powder
- 1 tsp chopped ginger
- 2 cup boiled rice
- 1 pinch salt
- 1 tbsp lemon juice

DIRECTIONS

1. In a pan, fry the mustard seeds, yellow split peas, and the black lentils for 3-4 minutes while stirring
2. Add the chili powder, chopped ginger and keep stirring
3. Add the boiled rice, salt, and lemon juice
4. Mix well, cook for 2 minutes and serve

Serves: *2*

Prep Time: *10*   Minutes

Cook Time: *20*   Minutes

Total Time: *30*   Minutes

INGREDIENTS

- 5 tbsp tahini
- 2 tbsp white miso paste
- 1 tbsp ginger
- 1 clove garlic
- 1 tbsp soy sauce
- 1 tbsp lemon juice
- 1 cup water
- 5 kale leaves
- 1 tbsp oil
- 1 sweet potato
- 3 tbsp boiled rice

DIRECTIONS

1. Combine tahini, miso paste, ginger, garlic, soy sauce, lemon juice and water in a blender for 3 minutes until smooth

2. Preheat oven to 375°F

3. Cut the potato in cubes and mix them with olive oil and salt

4. Put them in a baking dish and let them roast in the oven for 5-10 minutes until tender

5. Check them and stir to avoid sticking on the dish

6.

7. Tear the kale leaf into small pieces and mix them with 1 tbsp oil

8. Combine the cooked potato with kale and the first mixture and serve

Serves: **4**

Prep Time: **10** Minutes

Cook Time: **30** Minutes

Total Time: **40** Minutes

INGREDIENTS

- 1 cup split yellow mung beans
- 3 tbsp rice
- 5 cup water
- 1 cinnamon stick
- 2 tsp coriander
- 2 tsp turmeric
- a pinch salt
- a pinch pepper

DIRECTIONS

1. In a saucepan, place all the ingredients and water
2. Boil and cook on low heat until water is absorbed and keep stirring
3. Serve when ready

35

Serves: **4**

Prep Time: **10**   Minutes

Cook Time: **30**   Minutes

Total Time: **40**   Minutes

INGREDIENTS

- 2 cup brussels sprouts
- 1 onion
- 2 celery stalks
- 1 carrot
- 1 small cauliflower
- 1 tbsp parsley
- 1 tsp curry powder
- 2 tsp oil
- 1 garlic clove
- 2 tsp ground ginger
- 1 pinch salt
- 1 pinch pepper
- 3 tbsp coconut milk
- 3 cups vegetable soup

DIRECTIONS

1. In a pot, add 1 tbsp water and put the chopped onion, carrot, garlic, celery and spices and cook for 5-6 minutes

2. Add the vegetable soup and milk and boil

3. Simmer for 12-15 over low heat and start adding the brussels sprouts and cauliflower and, simmer for another 5-6 minutes

4. Place the mixture in a blender and blend for 2 minutes until smooth and add the parsley and serve

Serves: **6**

Prep Time: **10**   Minutes

Cook Time: **40**   Minutes

Total Time: **50**   Minutes

INGREDIENTS

- 1 cauliflower
- 1 can chickpeas
- 1 red pepper
- 1 onion
- 1 clove garlic
- 1 tsp turmeric
- 1 tsp coriander
- 1 pinch salt
- 1 pinch pepper
- 1 cup bread crumb

DIRECTIONS

1. Preheat oven to 370°F
2. Boil cauliflower until soft and fry the chopped onion along with the red pepper, chopped as well over low heat
3. Add garlic and pan for 2-3 minutes
4. In a bowl mash chickpeas and add the cauliflower and smash again
5. Add the other ingredients and mix well
6. Make medium balls out of the mixture and press between hands to make a patty
7. Fry the patties until brown and serve

Serves: *2*

Prep Time: *10*   Minutes

Cook Time: *25*   Minutes

Total Time: *35*   Minutes

INGREDIENTS

- 2 tbsp oil
- 1 tbsp curry powder
- a pinch salt
- 1 cup carrots
- 1 onion
- 2 cloves garlic
- 1 can plum tomatoes
- 1 cup coconut milk
- 3 tbsp tofu
- 1 cauliflower
- 1 tbsp lemon juice
- 2 tbs cilantro

DIRECTIONS

1. In a pan heat oil and add spices, chopped carrots, onion, garlic, and salt

2. Pan the ingredients for 9 minutes

3. Add coconut milk and tomatoes and boil, lower heat and cover with a lid and let it cook for 10 minutes

4. Transfer to a blender and blend until a creamy consistency

5. Sprinkle on top cilantro and serve warm

Serves: **10**

Prep Time: **5** Minutes

Cook Time: **10** Minutes

Total Time: **15** Minutes

INGREDIENTS

- 4 oz dried mango
- 4 oz cashew
- 1 oz oats
- 9 dried figs
- 1 tsp ground ginger
- 2 tbsp coconut oil
- a pinch salt
- coconut flakes

DIRECTIONS

1. **Put in a blender everything except the coconut flakes and blend for 4 minutes**
2. **Sprinkle coconut flakes on a plate**
3. **Form balls from the mixture and roll them on the plate with the coconut flakes and serve**

Serves: *2*

Prep Time: *10*   Minutes

Cook Time: *25*   Minutes

Total Time: *35*   Minutes

INGREDIENTS

- 2 sweet potatoes
- 5 tbsp oil
- 1 tsp turmeric
- 1 clove garlic
- 2 cups vegetable soup
- 2 tsp lemon juice
- 3 tsp parsley
- a pinch salt
- boiled egg
- 3 tbsp spinach
- 2 tbsp quinoa

DIRECTIONS

1. In a pan at medium heat, fry the sweet potato and add the turmeric, garlic and vegetable soup

2. Simmer until the soup is absorbed

3. Put the result in a bowl and smash, adding salt and pepper

4. Put lemon juice, 2 tsp oil, garlic, parsley, and salt in a blender to create the dressing

5. In a bowl, add the spinach and quinoa along with the mashed potatoes and pour over the dressing and serve

Serves: *2*

Prep Time: *20*   Minutes

Cook Time: *20*   Minutes

Total Time: *40*   Minutes

INGREDIENTS

- 3 tbsp coconut flakes
- 2 tbsp warm water
- 1 cup rice
- 3 tbsp mint leaves
- 2 tbsp cilantro
- 2 cloves garlic
- 1 green chili without seeds
- 1 tbsp butter or oil
- 1 onion
- 1 cinnamon stick
- 1 tsp cumin seeds
- 2 cups water

DIRECTIONS

1. Combine warm water with coconut flakes and stir. Let sit for 10 minutes and drain

2. Grind mint, cilantro, garlic, chili, and coconut until a paste has formed

3. In a saucepan, melt butter, add a cinnamon stick, cumin seeds and cook for 5-10 minutes, add chopped onions

4. Saute the onion and then add the paste and stir well for 3 more minutes

5. Add the rice and stir again for 3 minutes and then add 2 cups warm water and cover the saucepan with a lid and let it cook for 10 minutes and serve

Serves: *4*

Prep Time: *10*   Minutes

Cook Time: *60*   Minutes

Total Time: *70*   Minutes

INGREDIENTS

- 2 cups mung dal beans
- 1 cup rice
- 2 tbsp oil or butter
- 2 turmeric powder
- 2 tsp pepper
- 1 tsp coriander powder
- 3 cups spinach
- 3 cups carrots
- 3 cups kale
- 3 cups celery
- 1 cup cilantro

DIRECTIONS

1. Rinse the beans until the water runs clear
2. In a pan, heat oil and add spices

3. In the pan combine beans and rice and add vegetables and 8 cups water and let it cook for 60 minutes until it has a porridge consistency

4. Serve with cilantro sprinkled on top

Serves: *3*

Prep Time: *5*   Minutes

Cook Time: *25*   Minutes

Total Time: *30*   Minutes

INGREDIENTS

- **2 tbsp lentil**
- **4 tbsp rice**
- **4 cups water**
- **2 tsp cumin seeds**
- **2 tsp turmeric powder**
- **a pinch pepper**
- **2 tbsp oil**
- **a pinch salt**
- **2 green chilies**
- **2 tbsp cilantro**
- **2 tsp mustard seeds**

DIRECTIONS

1. **Combine rice with lentils**
2. **Boil them with 3 cups water until soft**

3. In a pan heat up the oil and put the mustard seeds until you hear them crackle

4. Add cumin seeds and chopped chilies and pan them for 1 minute and add turmeric and pepper. Set aside afterwards

5. Sprinkle salt over the lentils and rice and whisk

6. Mix the oil with spices and the lentils-rice together

7. Sprinkle cilantro on top and serve

Serves: 2
Prep Time: 2 Minutes

Cook Time: 15 Minutes

Total Time: 17 Minutes

INGREDIENTS

- 3 cups asparagus
- 3 carrots
- 1 cup yogurt
- 2 tbsp cucumber
- 2 tsp ground ginger
- 2 tsp cilantro
- a pinch turmeric
- a pinch pepper
- a pinch salt
- few peppermint leaves

DIRECTIONS

1. Boil or steam the asparagus and carrots until you can go through them with a fork

2. Juice the lemon add salt, honey, some peppermint leaves and blend them until smooth

3. In a bowl, add the yogurt, cucumber, ginger, cilantro, turmeric, pepper, salt, and mix. Set aside

4. Serve the asparagus and carrots with any of the sauces above

Serves: *3*

Prep Time: **5**   Minutes

Cook Time: **25**   Minutes

Total Time: *30*   Minutes

INGREDIENTS

- 3 red beets
- 3 carrots
- 4 tbsp coconut milk
- 2 tbsp oil
- 1 garlic clove
- 1 tsp cumin seeds
- a pinch turmeric
- a pinch salt
- a pinch pepper
- 1 onion

DIRECTIONS

1. In a frying pan, heat up the oil and saute the chopped onion for 4 minutes and add the chopped garlic and pan for a minute

2. Add the cumin seeds and cook for 2 minutes

3. Sprinkle pepper, turmeric, salt and cook for 1 minute

4. Put in the pan the chopped carrots and saute for 5 minutes

5. Before putting the beets, pre-boil them, peel them and chop them

6. Put the pre-boiled beets and let cook for another 5 minutes

7. Finally, pour the coconut milk and stir for 1 minute and add the cilantro

8. You can serve it with boiled rice

Serves: *2*

Prep Time: *10*   Minutes

Cook Time: *20*   Minutes

Total Time: *30*   Minutes

INGREDIENTS

- 1 cup rice
- 1 cup coconut milk
- 1 cup water
- a pinch salt
- 2 tsp coconut oil
- 1 tbsp chili paste
- 1 bunch kale
- 16 oz salmon

DIRECTIONS

1. Rinse rice in cold water and place in a pot with coconut milk, water, and salt

2. Let it boil stirring and then lower the heat to minimum and let it cook for 10-15 minutes

3. Heat the oven to 716°F

4. In a jar, add the melted coconut oil and the chili paste and shake well

5. Place kale on a baking sheet. Pour a little bit of the mixture and add the salmon

6. Pour the rest of the dressing and let it cook in the oven for 15-20 minutes

7. Serve with rice

Serves: *2*
Prep Time: *10*   Minutes

Cook Time: *30*   Minutes

Total Time: *40*   Minutes

INGREDIENTS

- 2 tsp oil
- 1 onion
- 3 celery sticks
- 1 sweet potato
- 3 tbsp chili powder
- a pinch ground cumin
- a pinch salt
- 15 oz beans
- 15 oz tomatoes
- 1 cup quinoa
- 1 lime
- 2 cups vegetable broth
- 3 carrots
- 1 avocado

DIRECTIONS

1. In a pot over medium heat warm up the oil and the chopped onion with celery for 5 minutes
2. In a bowl combine the chopped sweet potato, carrots, oil, chili, cumin and salt
3. Add the combination in the pot and stir
4. Add the beans, tomatoes, quinoa and the vegetable broth
5. Turn up the heat and let it boil
6. After, cover with a lid and let it covered for 30 minutes
7. Remove from the heat and let chill for 5 minutes
8. Serve with sliced avocado and squeeze the lime over it

Serves: 5
Prep Time: 5   Minutes

Cook Time: 25   Minutes

Total Time: 30   Minutes

INGREDIENTS

- 2 cups rice
- 4 cups nuts
- 1 cup fresh paneer
- 2 tbsp yogurt
- a pinch salt
- a pinch pepper
- butter
- flour
- 1 egg

DIRECTIONS

1. Boil the rice and blend the nuts
2. Combine all the ingredients, besides flour and make patties
3. Sprinkle flour on each patty and fry them in a frying pan with a little bit of butter
4. Serve it when ready

Serves: **2**

Prep Time: **5**   Minutes

Cook Time: **25**   Minutes

Total Time: **30**   Minutes

INGREDIENTS

- 2 tbsp oil
- 2 cloves garlic
- 1 small onion
- 1 cup chopped mushrooms
- 2 tbsp parsley
- 1 cup rice
- 5 tbsp white wine
- 2 cups any chopped greens you like
- a pinch pepper
- a pinch salt
- 1 cup vegetable broth

DIRECTIONS

1. In a pot over medium heat, add oil and the chopped garlic and onions and cook for 4-5 minutes
2. Add the chopped mushrooms with parsley and cook for 5 minutes
3. In another pot, bring to boil the vegetable broth and then reduce the heat
4. Add the rice and stir until you hear the rice crackle and then add the wine and stir until the liquid is absorbed, like 20-30 minutes
5. Add the chopped greens and add lemon juice while stirring
6. Serve the mushrooms with the rice

CURRY LENTIL WITH RICE AND CARROTS

Serves: *3*

Prep Time: *5*   Minutes

Cook Time: *55*   Minutes

Total Time: *60*   Minutes

INGREDIENTS

-    2 tbsp curry powder
-    2 tbsp butter
-    1 onion
-    2 cups lentils
-    2 tbsp salt
-    3 garlic cloves
-    2 tbsp yellow raisins
-    3 tbsp ground ginger
-    5 tbsp coconut milk
-    1 cup cilantro
-    1 cup rice
-    2 carrot
-    2 tomatoes

DIRECTIONS

1. Heat up the oven to 400°F and in a baking dish put the curry powder and roast it for 5 minutes and then add the butter the chopped onion and 2 cups lentils

2. Cover with water, add 2 tbsp salt sliced tomatoes, raisins, ground ginger and the chopped garlic cloves

3. Let cook with a lid on top for 35 minutes and then add the coconut milk, cilantro and stir well

4. Bring to a boil 1 cup water with coconut milk and a pinch of salt. Add 1 cup rice, cover with a lid and let cook for 20 minutes

5. Slice the carrots in a baking dish and put them in the oven with butter and let cook until golden brown

6. Serve the lentils with the rice and carrots

Serves: **1**

Prep Time: **5** Minutes

Cook Time: **5** Minutes

Total Time: **10** Minutes

INGREDIENTS

- 16 oz carrots
- 2 oranges
- 2 tbs dill
- 1 tsp ginger

DIRECTIONS

1. Over a bowl, peel off and cut the white pith and outer membrane from one orange
2. Grate 1 tsp of the peel and squeeze the juice from the second orange in a bowl and add the ginger and chopped carrots
3. Add the peeled orange and dill and mix well

Serves: **2**

Prep Time: **10**   Minutes

Cook Time: **20**   Minutes

Total Time: **30**   Minutes

INGREDIENTS

- 1 tbsp oil
- 1 onion
- 1 bell pepper
- 1 clove garlic
- 2 tomatoes
- 1 tsp ground cumin
- a pinch paprika
- 4 cups veggie broth
- 16 oz sea bass fillets
- 1 cup mushrooms
- 2 tbsp tahini
- 1 tbsp parsley
- 1 tbsp cilantro
- salt to taste

DIRECTIONS

1. In a pan over medium heat, put the oil and add the chopped onion and the diced bell pepper and pan for 5-10 minutes

2. Add the garlic and tomatoes and pan for 5 minutes

3. Sprinkle over the cumin and paprika powder and stir for 2 minutes

4. Pour the veggie broth and heat up and let it boil

5. Add the sliced mushrooms and the fish and wait for it to boil again and then low the heat and let it simmer for 5 minutes and serve

6. Mix in tahini the parsley, cilantro, salt and serve

Serves: *5*

Prep Time: *10*   Minutes

Cook Time: *50*   Minutes

Total Time: *60*   Minutes

INGREDIENTS

- 1 cup adzuki beans
- 2 onions
- 4 mushrooms
- 12 oz red potatoes
- 1 tbsp miso paste

DIRECTIONS

1. Soak the beans in cold water overnight and then drain the water

2. In a saucepan over medium-high heat, add the chopped onion, salt and cover it and let it cook for 6 minutes

3. Add the mushrooms and the beans and stir then add 4 cups water and let it boil

4. Reduce the heat to low and let simmer for 40 minutes

5. Fold in potatoes and cook for 10-15 minutes until tender

6. Take 1 cup water from the bean mixture and stir in the miso paste well and then pour it in the bean mixture, then stir and serve

67

Serves: 2

Prep Time: 5   Minutes

Cook Time: 15   Minutes

Total Time: 20   Minutes

INGREDIENTS

- 1 cup rice
- 1 cup broccoli
- 1 cup paneer
- 2 tbsp oil
- a pinch pepper
- 1 tsp lemon juice
- a pinch of ground ginger

DIRECTIONS

1. Boil the rice and chop the broccoli
2. Mix all the ingredients and serve

Serves: *4*

Prep Time: *10*   Minutes

Cook Time: *30*   Minutes

Total Time: *40*   Minutes

INGREDIENTS

- 16 oz chicken breasts
- salt to taste
- pepper to taste
- 6 garlic cloves
- 1 cup rice
- 3 tbsp parsley
- 3 tbsp lemon juice
- 2 cups water

DIRECTIONS

1. Massage the chicken breasts with salt and pepper and place in the oven at 350°F and add the rice and chopped garlic along with the lemon juice and water
2. Stir a few times and place in the oven for 30-40 minutes and serve with parsley on top

Serves:	*5*	
Prep Time:	*10*	Minutes
Cook Time:	*8 hrs*	Minutes
Total Time:	*8 hrs and 10 min*	Minutes

INGREDIENTS

- 2 onions
- 1 eggplant
- 4 zucchini
- 2 garlic cloves
- 2 bell peppers
- 6 tomatoes
- 1 tsp basil
- 2 tsp salt
- 2 pinch pepper
- 2 tbsp parsley
- 4 tbsp oil

DIRECTIONS

1. Slice the onions, eggplant, zucchini, garlic, bell pepper and tomatoes
2. Chop parsley

3. In a crockpot, layer half the veggies in this order: eggplant, onion, garlic, zucchini, green pepper, tomatoes, and repeat

4. Sprinkle salt, basil, pepper, and parsley on top and pour oil on top as well

5. Cover with a lid and cook on low for 8 hours and serve

Serves: 2

Prep Time: 5   Minutes

Cook Time: 25   Minutes

Total Time: 30   Minutes

INGREDIENTS

- 2 egg whites
- 1 tbsp cilantro
- 1 tsp lemon juice
- a pinch ground ginger
- 5 tbsp ground nuts
- 2 salmon fillets

DIRECTIONS

1. In a bowl, beat the egg whites, cilantro, lemon juice, ginger
2. Put the nuts in another bowl
3. Dip the salmon fillet in the egg mixture and then coat it in almonds
4. Place in a baking dish and bake at 840°F for 15-20 minutes and serve

Serves: *4*

Prep Time: *5*   Minutes

Cook Time: *15*   Minutes

Total Time: *20*   Minutes

INGREDIENTS

- 16 oz kale
- 2 cups tomatoes
- 1 cup onion
- 2 garlic cloves
- 1 pinch pepper
- 1 tsp salt

DIRECTIONS

1. Chop the tomatoes, onion, and garlic
2. Mix the tomatoes, onions, garlic, pepper, and salt in a saucepan and cook over medium-high heat for 5 minutes
3. Add the greens, stir and cook for 10-15 minutes
4. Serve when rea

Serves: *3*

Prep Time: *10*   Minutes

Cook Time: *4 hrs*   Minutes

Total Time: *4 hrs and 10 min*   Minutes

INGREDIENTS

- 3 chicken breasts
- 3 cups water
- 5 tbsp rice
- 3 tbsp quinoa
- salt to taste
- 28 oz tomatoes
- 1 celery stalk
- 2 carrots
- 1 onion
- 1 clove garlic

DIRECTIONS

1. Place chicken breasts, 2 cups water, rice, quinoa, chopped tomatoes and veggies in the crockpot
2. Cook on high for 2 hours and then stir and add salt, 1 cup water and cook again for 2 hours on medium
3. Serve when ready

Serves: *3*

Prep Time: *5*   Minutes

Cook Time: *15*   Minutes

Total Time: *20*   Minutes

INGREDIENTS

- 32 oz kale
- 1 tbsp garlic
- 5 tbsp oil
- 3 tbsp dried goji

DIRECTIONS

1. Boil kale in a pot then put it in cold water and drain
2. Fry garlic over medium heat while stirring and then add kale, goji, salt, pepper and cook for 5-6 minutes
3. Serve warm

Serves: *3*

Prep Time: *10*   Minutes

Cook Time: *15*   Minutes

Total Time: *25*   Minutes

INGREDIENTS

- 1 cup orzo
- salt to taste
- 4 cups water
- 32 oz tomatoes
- 1 onion
- 1 tsp cinnamon powder
- 1 clove garlic
- 2 tbsp oil
- 1 tbsp basil

DIRECTIONS

1. In a pot boil, the orzo with salt and 4 cups water then set aside
2. In a pot over medium heat cook tomatoes, chopped onion, cinnamon powder, chopped garlic, salt, oil and cook while stirring for 10-15 minutes
3. Serve the orzo with spiced tomato sauce with basil on top

Serves: 2

Prep Time: 5   Minutes

Cook Time: 30   Minutes

Total Time: 35   Minutes

INGREDIENTS

- 1 cup rice
- 2 fennel bulbs
- 1 celery stalk
- 1 red pepper
- 2 tbsp oil
- 2 tbsp lemon juice
- 2 tbsp mint
- 2 tbsp parsley
- a pinch salt
- a pinch pepper

DIRECTIONS

1. Put rice in a bowl and pour water and soak in for 25-30 minutes
2. Drain the rice and then steam with chopped pepper and set aside
3. Combine all ingredients in a bowl and serve

Serves: **2**

Prep Time: **10**   Minutes

Cook Time: **20**   Minutes

Total Time: **30**   Minutes

INGREDIENTS

- 4 oz rice
- 1 avocado
- 1 tomato
- 2 tbsp oil
- 2 tsp soy sauce
- 2 garlic clove
- 1 tsp cilantro
- a pinch red pepper seeds

DIRECTIONS

1. Boil the rice, drain it and set aside
2. In a bowl add the sliced avocado, chopped tomatoes, oil, soy sauce, chopped garlic, rep pepper seeds and mix well
3. Combine the rice with the avocado mixture and serve with cilantro on top

78

Serves: **3**

Prep Time: **10**   Minutes

Cook Time: **30**   Minutes

Total Time: **40**   Minutes

INGREDIENTS

- **a pinch ground coriander**
- **a pinch paprika**
- **a pinch cinnamon**
- **a pinch pepper**
- **2 tbsp oil**
- **2 carrots**
- **1 bell pepper**
- **1 fennel bulb**
- **1 zucchini**
- **1 squash**
- **2 tomatoes**
- **1 cup peas**
- **2 cups veggie broth**
- **1 cup couscous**
- **2 tbsp cilantro**

DIRECTIONS

79

1. In a pan, heat oil and pan the chopped carrots, bell pepper, add the sliced fennel, zucchini, squash, tomatoes, spices and cook for 5-10 minutes and stir well

2. Pour in veggie broth and bring it to a boil, then let it simmer for 20 minutes

3. In a pot, bring to a boil 1 cup water and add couscous then let it simmer or 5 minutes

4. Combine the couscous with the vegetables and broth and serve

Serves: **2**
Prep Time: **5**   Minutes

Cook Time: **25**   Minutes

Total Time: **30**   Minutes

INGREDIENTS

- 1 onion
- 1 tsp oil
- 1 clove garlic
- a pinch cinnamon
- 16 oz kale
- 1 cup veggie broth
- a pinch salt
- a pinch pepper
- 1 tbsp chives

DIRECTIONS

1. In a frying pan heat olive oil and fry onion for 5 minutes
2. Add the chopped garlic, cinnamon and cook for 2 more minutes
3. Add the kale and veggie broth and let cook for 10-15 minutes covered
4. Sprinkle salt, pepper, chives and serve

Serves: 2

Prep Time: 5   Minutes

Cook Time: 5   Minutes

Total Time: *10*   Minutes

INGREDIENTS

- 1 tsp chili seeds
- 3 cups grates carrots
- 3 tbsp chopped figs
- 1 tbsp ground ginger
- 2 tbsp lemon juice
- 2 tbsp orange juice
- a pinch cinnamon powder
- a pinch salt

DIRECTIONS

1. In a pan, heat olive oil, add the carrots and fry for 30 seconds
2. Transfer to a bowl
3. Add all the rest of the ingredients and mix well and serve

Serves: *4*

Prep Time: *15*   Minutes

Cook Time: *65*   Minutes

Total Time: *80*   Minutes

INGREDIENTS

- 1 squash
- 2 tbsp butter
- 1 cup rice
- 1 tsp ground ginger
- 3 tbsp celery
- 3 tbsp carrots
- 3 tbsp nuts
- 3 tbsp raisins
- a pinch cinnamon
- a pinch pepper
- a pinch salt

DIRECTIONS

1. Preheat the oven to 350°F
2. Cut in half lengthwise the squash and bake for 40 minutes
3. Boil the rice and simmer for 20-25 minutes

4. In a pan, melt butter and fry the chopped celery, carrots, nuts, ground ginger, and raisins

5. Place the mixture into the rice bowl

6. Scoop out the centers from squash

7. With a fork and butter, mash it until you get to the squash's shell

8. Add the rice, mix and serve

Serves: *4*

Prep Time: *10* Minutes

Cook Time: *30* Minutes

Total Time: *40* Minutes

INGREDIENTS

- 2 cups yogurt
- a pinch salt
- a pinch pepper
- 2 tbsp chopped mint
- 2 cucumbers

DIRECTIONS

1. Peel the cucumber and chop it
2. Combiner all the ingredients and serve

Serves: *5*

Prep Time: *10*   Minutes

Cook Time: *30*   Minutes

Total Time: *40*   Minutes

INGREDIENTS

- 3 cups water
- 1 cup rice
- 5 tbsp quinoa
- 3 tbsp oats
- 3 tbsp nuts
- 1 onion
- 2 tbsp butter
- pepper
- 1 tsp coriander
- 2 tbsp parsley
- 3 tbsp soy sauce

DIRECTIONS

1. Fry the chopped onion in oil until golden brown
2. Add the crushed nuts and pepper, coriander and cook for 1 minute

3.   Add the quinoa, rice, water and soy sauce

4.   Simmer on low heat for 15 minutes covered

5.   After, stir in the oats and parsley

6.   Create burger patties and bake for 15 minutes at 400°F

7.   Serve when ready

AMAZING ALMOND PUDDING

Serves: 3

Prep Time: *3 hrs*   Minutes

Cook Time: *30*   Minutes

Total Time: *3 hrs 30 min*   Minutes

INGREDIENTS

- 5 tbsp almonds
- 10 oz hot water
- 1 cup milk
- 5 tbsp cream
- 1 tbsp flour
- 3 tbsp sugar

DIRECTIONS

1. Place the almonds in water and soak for 2-3 hours
2. Blend almonds with water and then add half of the milk
3. Boil the remaining milk and cream together and stir constantly
4. Add flour and the almond mixture and reduce the heat to low
5. Cook for 30 minutes and serve when ready

Serves: **6**

Prep Time: **10** Minutes

Cook Time: **40** Minutes

Total Time: **50** Minutes

INGREDIENTS

- 4 oz butter
- 2 cup flour
- 2 tsp baking powder
- 10 oz buttermilk
- 1 cup sugar
- 10 oz water
- 2 pinch baking soda
- 1 tsp cinnamon
- 2 pinch salt

DIRECTIONS

1. Preheat the oven to 350°F
2. Butter and flour lightly a baking dish
3. Mix butter and sugar until creamy
4. Combine the dry ingredients and mix with the cream

5. Mix water with buttermilk and pour over the mix and dry ingredients and whisk

6. Spoon the mixture into a baking dish

7. In a bowl, mix sugar and flour then cut the butter in and mix it then sprinkle over the baking dish

8. Bake for 40 minutes and serve warm

Serves: **5**

Prep Time: **5**   Minutes

Cook Time: **60**   Minutes

Total Time: **65**   Minutes

INGREDIENTS

- 2 cups grated carrots
- 3 tbsp butter
- 6 cup milk
- 10 oz sugar
- a pinch cinnamon
- 5 tbsp heavy cream
- 1 cup chopped nuts

DIRECTIONS

1. In a pan, melt butter, add the carrots and fry for 7 minutes
2. Add the milk and let it boil while stirring
3. Reduce the heat and let cook for 30 minutes
4. Add sugar and cook for 20 more minutes and stir
5. Add the heavy cream and cinnamon and let cook for 5 minutes then remove from heat
6. Serve with nuts

Serves: **8**

Prep Time: **5** Minutes

Cook Time: **15** Minutes

Total Time: **20** Minutes

INGREDIENTS

- 4 oz butter
- 5 tbsp sugar
- 2 eggs
- 3 tbsp yogurt
- 2 pinch baking soda
- 1 tsp baking powder
- 1 cup oats
- 2 cups flour

DIRECTIONS

1. In a bowl, add all the ingredients except the flour
2. Mix well, add flour slowly and stir
3. Preheat the oven to 350°F and roll the dough into balls
4. Place each ball on a baking sheet, bake for 15 minutes and serve

Serves: *4*

Prep Time: *10*   Minutes

Cook Time: *10*   Minutes

Total Time: *20*   Minutes

INGREDIENTS

- 2 bananas
- 2 tbsp butter
- a pinch salt
- a pinch pepper
- a pinch cumin
- a pinch turmeric

DIRECTIONS

1. Peel the bananas and slice them
2. Heat up butter in a pan and place the slices and let cook for 3 minutes then flip and again 3 minutes
3. Remove the slices and place them on a paper towel to remove excess oil and serve

Serves: *4*

Prep Time: *10*   Minutes

Cook Time: *15*   Minutes

Total Time: *25*   Minutes

INGREDIENTS

- 5 sweet potatoes
- 4 tbsp butter
- 1 cup sugar
- 1 tsp cinnamon

DIRECTIONS

1. Peel off, boil and mash the potatoes
2. Heat up butter in a saucepan until hot
3. Add the mashed potatoes and stir for 5 minutes
4. Add sugar, stir and let it cook for 5 minutes
5. Add the cinnamon, stir and remove from heat and serve

Serves: *4*
Prep Time: *5*   Minutes

Cook Time: *30*   Minutes

Total Time: *35*   Minutes

INGREDIENTS

- 15 oz apricot halves
- 6 whole allspice
- 3 tbsp butter
- a pinch cinnamon
- 4 oz water
- 1 lemon
- 2 tbsp peppermint leaves

DIRECTIONS

1. Squeeze the lemon
2. Combine all the ingredients except the apricots in a saucepan and bring to a boil
3. Reduce the heat and simmer for 10-12 minutes
4. Add the fruits and stir well
5. Cover and let sit for 30 minutes, serve when ready

Serves: *3*

Prep Time: *10*   Minutes

Cook Time: *15*   Minutes

Total Time: *25*   Minutes

INGREDIENTS

- 2 cups raisins
- 2 cups cashew
- 2 tbsp butter
- 1 cup water
- 1 tbsp rose water
- 1 cup sugar
- 1 cup oats

DIRECTIONS

1. Fry the raisins and cashews in oil and set aside
2. Boil water and after it cools, add the rose water
3. In a saucepan, combine the oats and butter and stir over medium heat for 4 minutes
4. Add sugar and mix well
5. Add the rose water and the cashew and raisins
6. Keep stirring for 1 minute and serve after cooling down

Serves: *3*

Prep Time: *5*   Minutes

Cook Time: *45*   Minutes

Total Time: *50*   Minutes

INGREDIENTS

- 2 cups rice
- 5 tbsp raisins
- 2 cinnamon sticks
- 1 tsp butter
- 2 tbsp sugar
- 2 cups milk

DIRECTIONS

1. In a pot, add the rice and milk and cook on low heat and stir occasionally
2. Add the cinnamon sticks and cook for 15 minutes
3. Add raisins and stir
4. Add butter and cook for 30 minutes
5. Serve when ready

Serves: **4**

Prep Time: **5** Minutes

Cook Time: **55** Minutes

Total Time: **60** Minutes

INGREDIENTS

- 3 pears
- lemon juice from 1 lemon
- 4 tbsp ginger
- 1 cup flour
- 1 cup oats
- 3 tbsp sugar
- 3 tbsp butter

DIRECTIONS

1. In a saucepan combine the peeled and chopped pears with the lemon juice and ginger and let cook on low heat for 15 minutes
2. In a bowl mix the rest of the ingredients
3. Place the first half of the mixture in the baking dish
4. Pour over the pear mixture
5. Sprinkle on top the rest of the crumb and bake for 40 minutes at 350°F and serve

Serves: *1*

Prep Time: *5*   Minutes

Cook Time: *5*   Minutes

Total Time: *10*   Minutes

INGREDIENTS

- 5 figs
- 1 cup milk
- a pinch cinnamon

DIRECTIONS

1. In a blender place all ingredients and blend until smooth
2. Pour the smoothie in a glass and serve

Serves: *1*

Prep Time: *5*   Minutes

Cook Time: *5*   Minutes

Total Time: *10*   Minutes

INGREDIENTS

- orange juice
- 1 handful blueberries
- 1 handful cranberries
- 1 handful raspberries
- 1 kiwi
- 1 peach

DIRECTIONS

1. In a blender place all ingredients and blend until smooth
2. Pour the smoothie in a glass and serve

Serves: 2

Prep Time: 5   Minutes

Cook Time: 5   Minutes

Total Time: 10   Minutes

INGREDIENTS

- 1 cup cold water
- 1 cucumber
- 3 celery stalks
- 1 tbsp cilantro
- 1 tbsp parsley
- juice a lemon

DIRECTIONS

1. Peel the cucumber and chop it
2. In a blender place all ingredients and blend until smooth
3. Pour the smoothie in a glass and serve

Serves: *1*

Prep Time: *5*   Minutes

Cook Time: *5*   Minutes

Total Time: *10*   Minutes

INGREDIENTS

- 2 cups milk
- 1 mango

DIRECTIONS

1. In a blender place all ingredients and blend until smooth
2. Pour the smoothie in a glass and serve

Serves: **1**

Prep Time: **5** Minutes

Cook Time: **5** Minutes

Total Time: **10** Minutes

INGREDIENTS

- 2 cups chopped honeydew
- 1 cup chopped cucumber
- 10 mint leaves
- 3 tbsp lemon juice
- 1 tsp honey

DIRECTIONS

1. In a blender place all ingredients and blend until smooth
2. Pour the smoothie in a glass and serve

Serves: *1*

Prep Time: *5*   Minutes

Cook Time: *5*   Minutes

Total Time: *10*   Minutes

INGREDIENTS

- 1 cup milk
- 10 oz berries
- 3 tbsp coconut water
- 1 tsp any syrup you like

DIRECTIONS

1. In a blender place all ingredients and blend until smooth
2. Pour the smoothie in a glass and serve

Serves: *1*

Prep Time: *5*   Minutes

Cook Time: *5*   Minutes

Total Time: *10* Minutes

INGREDIENTS

- 1 cup milk
- 4 dates
- a pinch cinnamon

DIRECTIONS

1. In a blender place all ingredients and blend until smooth
2. Pour the smoothie in a glass and serve

Serves: *1*

Prep Time: *5*   Minutes

Cook Time: *5*   Minutes

Total Time: *10*   Minutes

INGREDIENTS

- half baked avocado
- 5 tbsp coconut milk
- 1 cup chopped pineapple
- 5 kale leaves
- 1 tsp maple syrup
- a pinch of salt

DIRECTIONS

1. In a blender place all ingredients and blend until smooth
2. Pour the smoothie in a glass and serve

Serves: *1*

Prep Time: **5**   Minutes

Cook Time: **5**   Minutes

Total Time: ***10***   Minutes

INGREDIENTS

- 1 coconut
- 3 figs
- 2 pinches cinnamon

DIRECTIONS

1. In a blender place all ingredients and blend until smooth
2. Pour the smoothie in a glass and serve

Serves: *1*

Prep Time: **5**   Minutes

Cook Time: **5**   Minutes

Total Time: ***10***   Minutes

INGREDIENTS

- 1 cup almond milk
- 5 tbsp chopped mango
- 1 banana
- 1 tbsp coconut oil
- 3 pinches turmeric
- 3 pinches cinnamon
- 3 pinches ginger
- a pinch salt
- a pinch pepper
- 1 tsp honey

DIRECTIONS

1. In a blender place all ingredients and blend until smooth
2. Pour the smoothie in a glass and serve

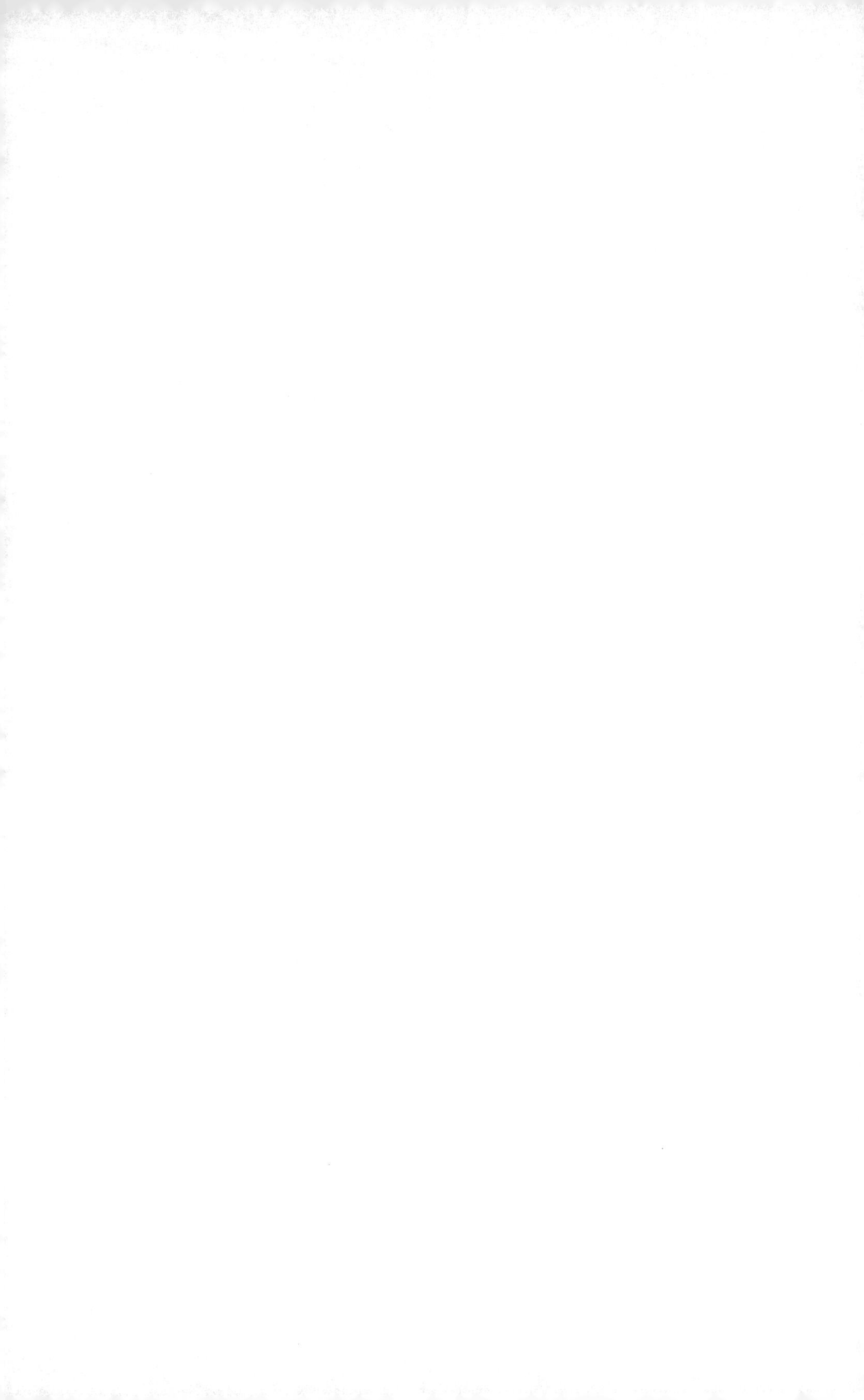